BEI GRIN MACHT SICH IHR WISSEN BEZAHLT

- Wir veröffentlichen Ihre Hausarbeit,
  Bachelor- und Masterarbeit

- Ihr eigenes eBook und Buch -
  weltweit in allen wichtigen Shops

- Verdienen Sie an jedem Verkauf

Jetzt bei www.GRIN.com hochladen und kostenlos publizieren

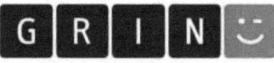

Productive and reproductive Performance of indigenous Beef Cattle in Ethiopia

Tajudin Denur

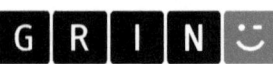

Bibliografische Information der Deutschen Nationalbibliothek:

Die Deutsche Nationalbibliothek verzeichnet diese Publikation in der Deutschen Nationalbibliografie; detaillierte bibliografische Daten sind im Internet über http://dnb.d-nb.de abrufbar.

ISBN: 9783346338266
Dieses Buch ist auch als E-Book erhältlich.

© GRIN Publishing GmbH
Nymphenburger Straße 86
80636 München

Druck und Bindung: Books on Demand GmbH, Norderstedt Germany
Gedruckt auf säurefreiem Papier aus verantwortungsvollen Quellen

Das vorliegende Werk wurde sorgfältig erarbeitet. Dennoch übernehmen Autoren und Verlag für die Richtigkeit von Angaben, Hinweisen, Links und Ratschlägen sowie eventuelle Druckfehler keine Haftung.

Das Buch bei GRIN: https://www.grin.com/document/982809

SCHOOL OF GRADUATE STUDIES

COLLEGE OF AGRICULTURAL SCIENCE

DEPARTEMENT OF ANIMAL SCIENCE

REVIEW ON

PRODUCTIVE AND REPRODUCTIVE PERFORMANCE OF BEEF

CATTLE IN ETHIOPIA

A TERM PAPER FOR THE COURSE APPLIED ANIMAL BREEDING SUBMITTED TO

DEPARTMENT OF ANIMAL SCIENCES

BY: TAJUDIN

JANUARY, 2020

ARBAMINCH, ETHIOPIA

Table of Contents

LIST OF TABLES II

ABBREVIATIONS / ACRONYMS III

EXECUTIVE SUMMARY V

1.   INTRODUCTION 1

2.   LITRATURE REVIEW 4

    2.1.   Indigenous Cattle Breeds of Ethiopia 4

    2.2.   Reproductive performance of indigenous Ethiopian cattle 4

        2.2.1.   Age at first calving (AFC): 4

        2.2.2.   Calving interval (CI): 5

        2.2.3.   Number of services per-conception (NSPC): 7

        2.2.4.   Days open (DO): 8

        2.2.5.   Age at first service (AFS) 9

    2.3.   Growth performance of indigenous Ethiopian cattle 10

        2.3.1.   Birth weight and weights at different ages 11

        2.3.2.   Average daily body weight gain (ADG) 12

        2.3.3.   Carcass yield performance of indigenous Ethiopian cattle 13

3.   CONCLUSION AND RECOMMENDATION 18

REFERENCES 20

LIST OF TABLES

Table 1 Summary of age at first calving and calving interval (in month) of Ethiopian Indigenous breeds 7

Table 2 Summary of age at first calving, days open and number of service per conception of Ethiopian Indigenous breeds 9

Table 3 Birth weight and weight at different age of indigenous breed of Ethiopia 11

Table 4 Comparison between average body weight gain of boran and kereyu senga breeds with in different ages 12

Table 5 Literature of carcass characteristics of some Ethiopian beef cattle breeds 13

Table 6 Carcass yield performance of the two Ethiopian indigenous cattle breed 14

Table 7 Effects of cattle of age and breed on carcass characteristics. 15

ABBREVIATIONS / ACRONYMS

Age at first calving	AFC
Age at first service	AFS
Average daily body weight gain	ADG
Birth weight	BWT
Calving interval	CI
Calving-to-conception interval	CCI
Central Statistical Agency	CSA
Days open	DO
Domestic Animal Diversity Information System	DADIS
Domestic Animal Genetic Resources Information System	DAGRIS
Ethiopian Institute of Biodiversity Conservation	EIBC
Ethiopia Strategy Support Program II	ESSP II
Food and Agriculture Organization	FAO
Gram	g
Improving Productivity and Market Success	IPMS
Kilo gram	Kg
Mature weight	MWT
Ministry of Agriculture	MOA
Ministry of Agriculture and Rural Development	MoARD
Number of services per-conception	NSPC

Slaughtering weight	SWT
United States Department of Agriculture	USDA
Weaning weight	WWT
Yearling weight	YWT

EXECUTIVE SUMMARY

The aim of this review is to summarize the Productive and reproductive performance of different indigenous cattle breeds under farmer's management practices. Ethiopia is the home of large numbers of livestock due to having varied and extensive agro-ecological zones. From the total annual milk produced cattle milk, is the most prominent compared to other livestock species in Ethiopia. And also from the total annual meat produced cattle meat is the most prominent compared to other livestock species in Ethiopia. Numerous finding showed that calving interval, age at first calving, age at first service, number of service per conception and days open are one of the major measures of reproductive performance parameters for beef cattle production. Weight at different ages (including birth weight, weaning weight, 3 month weight, 6 month weight and yearling weight), meat yield, growth rate and carcass yield are one of the major measures of productive performance parameters for beef cattle production. Different report indicated that productive and reproductive performances of our indigenous cattle are very poor due to varied factors; the causes for low performances of beef cattle were genetic and environmental factors like feeding, housing and health care. In Ethiopia most of (98.20%) cattle breeds are local breeds the remaining (1.8%) are hybrid and exotic breeds. Then, the genetic performances of these breeds are poor, even though they have good adaptation in harsh environmental conditions. So, training and awareness creation should be given particularly to the farmers on major management practices like feeding, housing and health care and genetic improvement strategies should planned and practiced.

Keywords: Beef, Ethiopia, Productive performance, Management, Reproductive performance, Calving interval, birth weight, Carcass weight

1. INTRODUCTION

Agricultural sector of Ethiopia accounts for about 42% of the GDP, employs about 85% of the labor force, and contributes around 90% of the total export earnings of the country. The sector is dominated by over 15 million smallholders producing about 95% of the national agricultural production. Hence, the overall economy of the country and the food security of the majority of the population depend on smallholder agriculture (CSA, 2015, 2016). Ethiopia is rich in livestock population that owned 59.5 million cattle, 30.7 million sheep, 30.2 million goats and 59.5 million chickens (CSA, 2016, 2017). Ethiopia is believed to have the largest livestock population in Africa (CSA, 2017). The varied and extensive agro ecological zones and the importance of livestock in livelihood strategies make Ethiopia home to large numbers of livestock. Ethiopia has 59,486,667 cattle (CSA, 2017) and out of this total cattle population, the female cattle constitute about 55.5 percent and the remaining 44.5 percent are male cattle. Eighty-three percent of all milk produced in Ethiopia comes from cattle with the remainder coming from goats and camels (MoARD, 2007). Which is lower than the report of CSA (2011) and CSA (2017) cows contribute to about 95% and 94.6 % of the total annual milk produced compared to other livestock species, respectively.

Despite the largest cattle population in Ethiopia productive and reproductive performances are very poor (Yosefe et al., 2003; Belay et al., 2012 and Melku et al., 2016). Similarly, Niraj et al. (2014b) and Nibret et al. (2014) reported that reproductive performance of indigenous cows was found to be less than the optimum values desirable for profitable milk production in different parts of Ethiopia. According to Belay et al., (2012) the cause for low performances of indigenous cattle might be genetic and environmental factors like feed shortage, low level of management, lack of access to land, disease, lack of proper poor breeding management such as lack of accurate heat detection and timely insemination might have contributed considerably to long days open (postpartum anestrous), late age at first calving, long calving interval, short lactation length and low milk production.

Major livestock species were imported to enhance livestock productivity of Ethiopia through crossbreeding. Accordingly, the number of breeds of cattle, sheep, goat and chicken imported so far to Ethiopia are 7, 7, 3, and 14, respectively (EIBC, 2012). Cattle are the most important species followed by goats, camels, and sheep in the pastoral livestock production system, and are source

1

of food in the form of milk, meat and blood, and source of other products such as fiber and hides (FAO, 2009). Cattle herds are much larger in the pastoral areas and average about 75 head in Borena, Ethiopia. In the mixed farming areas, herds are much smaller being 5.7 head in East Harerghe, 8.6 in Illubabor and 11.8 in the central highlands (MoARD, 2007). In mixed farming system, cattle provide draught power and manure for cropland fertilization beside to milk production (Agajie *et al.*, 2002), whereas the purpose of keeping cattle in pastoral production system is for breeding and selling, in agro pastoral production system for meat and draught power and in highland mixed crop-livestock production is for draught power and sale of culls (MoARD, 2007).

A more recent report indicated that 98.20% of the total cattle population in Ethiopia are local breeds while hybrid and exotic breeds accounted for about 1.62 and 0.18%, respectively (CSA, 2016/2017). FAO (1993) reported that cow milk constitutes 83.4% of the total milk produced in Ethiopia and CSA (2008/09) also indicated that cattle have the largest contribution (81.2%) of the total national annual milk output. CSA (2014/2015) report on milk utilization indicated that 46.36% of the total annual milk production was used for household consumption, 5.98% was sold, only 0.33% was used for wages in kind and the rest 43.33% was used for other products (could be for the production of butter, Cheese, and others). CSA (2014/15) also reported on beef cattle utilization in that 52.93% of the total annual production was used for household consumption, 33.18% was used sold, 0.71% was paid for wages in kind and 13.18% was used for other products. Indigenous livestock breeds whose adaptive traits permit survival and reproduction under the harsh climatic, nutritional and management conditions typically associated with resource-poor livestock keepers have been shown to outperform crossbreeds under such circumstances (Ayalew *et al.*, 2003). The annual contribution of ruminants to meat production in Ethiopia is estimated at over 3.2 million tones, representing over 72% of the total meat production. Cattle meat accounts for over 70% of the total red meat production and over 50% of the total meat output in Sub-Saharan Africa (EARO, 1999).

The productivity of cattle depends largely on their reproductive performance. Reproduction is an indicator of reproductive efficiency and the rate of genetic progress in both selection and crossbreeding programs particularly in dairy and beef production (Nuraddis, 2011). Currently in Ethiopia there are 409,869 beef cattle and last year 69,830 beef cattle were slaughtered for

2

consumption and export purpose (CSA, 2016). Cattle contribute about 80% of GDP that come from livestock (Tefera, 2011). Cattle in Ethiopia produced about 0.331 million tons of meat annually (CSA, 2008). Average carcass weight of cattle was 108 kg/head (Negassa *et al.*, 2011), while Ethiopians consume about 8 kg of meat per capita annually which is far less than what is consumed in developing countries (Betru and Kawashima, 2009).

Beef consumers desire disease free animal, cuts of beef that are lean, nutritious and possess desirable eating characteristics such as tenderness, juiciness, color, texture and flavor. Several factors affect these carcass characteristics such as breed, age of the animal and feed. Even though, little work has been done concerning carcass and growth evaluation in Ethiopia (Tesfaye *et al.*1993; Nega *et al* 2002) that were accomplished by different institutions, which are available related to factors affecting carcass characteristics. There are different cattle populations in the country, however, the national cattle characterization work of each cattle population is not well summarized and the current state of knowledge on all indigenous cattle is not known. Moreover, it is obvious and many times reported that cattle productivity in Ethiopia is extremely low. This low cattle productivity is due to different cattle production challenges. Therefore, it is essential to know cattle challenges and opportunities at national level to be an input in the future research and development works With this number of livestock population Ethiopia stand first in Africa and 10th in the world. However, the production and productivity of this livestock is not commensurate with the number. Therefore, the objective of this paper is to review the productive and reproductive performances of indigenous beef cattle of Ethiopia.

2. LITRATURE REVIEW

2.1. Indigenous Cattle Breeds of Ethiopia

FAO (2005) reported that cattle contribute 40% of the annual agricultural output and 15% of the total gross domestic product. Ethiopia has 59.5 million heads of cattle (CSA, 2016/2017). Ethiopian Institute of Biodiversity Conservation (EIBC) (2004) reported that Sheko, Fogera, Begait and Boran cattle populations were at decreasing trend. According to Rege (1999), two Ethiopian indigenous cattle breeds (Arsi-Sanga and Kuri) are already reported as extinct. DAGRIS (Access date: November 21/2017) report indicated that the current number of indigenous cattle breeds of Ethiopia are 37. CSA (2016/2017) reported that about 98.2% of the total cattle population was indigenous cattle population, 1.62% of the cattle populations in Ethiopia were crossbred and 0.18% exotic cattle.

2.2. Reproductive performance of indigenous Ethiopian cattle

Reproductive traits describe the animal's ability to conceive, calve down and suckle the calf to weaning successfully (Davis, 1993); these traits are important since they affect the herd size. Reproductive performance is commonly evaluated by analyzing female reproductive traits (Aynalem *et al.*, 2011) of a combination of many traits (Olawumi and Salako, 2010). Reproduction is an indicator of reproductive efficiency and the rate of genetic progress in both selection and crossbreeding programs particularly in dairy and beef production (Mukassa Mugerewa and Azage, 1991). High reproductive efficiency is necessary for efficient milk production and has an important influence on herd profitability (Pryce *et al.*, 2004). Reproductive efficiency is expressed by the extent of reduction of reproductive wastage and it affects lifetime milk and meat production (Nuraddis, 2011). The main indicators that would be considered in assessing reproductive performance are age at puberty, age at first calving, calving interval, days open and number of services per conception (Yifat, 2009; Habtamu *et al.*, 2010; Aynalem *et al.*, 2011; Demissu *et al.*, 2013).

2.2.1. Age at first calving (AFC):

Age at first calving is the period between birth and first calving and influences both the productive and reproductive life of the female, directly through its effect on her lifetime calf crop and milk production and indirectly through its influence on the cost invested for up-bringing (Gebrekidan *et al.*, 2012). Age at first calving is closely related to the rearing intensity, and in a breeding program has impact on generation interval and response to selection. It is affected by nutrition, year and month of birth (Kelay, 2002). AFC obtained in this review for Horro breeds was between 50 to 58.08±0.07 months. Where as AFC obtained in this review for Boran breed was between 22.6 to 58.8. But, AFC obtained in this review for Fogera breed was between 50.8±0.36 to 63 months. And AFC obtained in this review for Arsi breed was between 32.8 to 55.4±0.7 months. However, AFC obtained in this review for Bagait breed was between 48.68±0.16 to 60 months. But the reviewed result obtained for breed of shorter AFC indicates that the breed can calve at younger age than others. Researchers stated that year of birth had significant effect on the age at first calving. Which means age at first calving increased as year goes (Melaku *et al.*2011; Giday, Y. E 2001, Addisu B. 1999). The longer average age at first calving reported for indigenous cattle might be associated with scarcity of feed and shortage of water for the long dry season of the year in the study area. Brief information is summarized in the table below (table 1).

2.2.2. Calving interval (CI):

It is the period between successive parturitions and is a function of postpartum anestrus period (from calving to first estrus), service period (first postpartum estrus to conception) and gestation length (Tewodros, 2008). CI has two components: 1) calving-to-conception interval (CCI) or days open, which is considered to be the most important component determining the length of the calving interval, and 2) gestation length, which is more or less constant, varying slightly due to breed, calf sex, litter size, dam age, year and month of calving, and little can be done to significantly manipulate the gestation length (Mukasa-Mugerwa *et al.*, 1991). The CCI itself is influenced by cow and management/environment-related factors, such as method and efficiency of heat detection, type and efficiency of breeding service and the ability of the cow to resume regular ovarian cyclicity after calving, display an overt heat signs, and conceive with the given service. The gap between two successive calving is called calving interval (Mulugeta and Belayeneh, 2013). Calving interval is an important factor in measuring the breeding efficiency and directly correlates with the economics of milk production. Reproduction in dairy cows with regular and shorter calving interval (365-420 days) is a key feature for the rapid multiplication of the breeding stocks. Estimates of calving interval in zebu cattle range from 12.2 to 26.6 months (Mukassa-Mugrewa, 1989; Gebrekidan *et al.*, 2012). Nutritional conditions that vary seasonally and yearly and parity (Prabhakar and Addisu, 2004) have major effect on calving interval

5

(Hailemariam and Kassa, 1994). The effectiveness of estrus detection and conception rate has a great impact on the calving interval. Calving interval is probably the best indicator of cattle reproductive efficiency. It is fertility traits that can be used in selection programs to minimize the negative effects that selection for production have on fertility (Mostert *et al.*, 2010).

CI obtained in this review for Boran breed was between 11.8 to 20.7 months. Whereas CI obtained in this review for Fogera breed was between 17.5 to 37 months. And also CI obtained in this review for Horro breed was between 12 to 21.08± 0.3 months. But the values obtained in this review for Boran breed was slightly comparable with Horro breed. As I reviewed that the result obtained from Horro and Boran breed was shorter than any of others indigenous breed. This indicated that Horro and Boran breed can calve at short time than others. This is because of that Short CI was reported for cows which calved during the short rainy season than those calved during dry and long rainy season. This could be due to the availability of adequate pasture during this and the coming main rainy season which may enable the cow in good condition during and after calving for re-conception in the following breeding season. On the contrary, cows calved during the main rainy season had the longest CI. This might be because of lack of green pasture and supplementary feed in the coming dry season and due to the incidence of skin disease (Demodex) during main rainy season. Researchers stated that year of birth had significant effect on the calving interval. However, there was no clear trend of effect of year (Melaku *et al.*2011; Giday, Y.E 2001, Addisu B. 1999). Cattles having the longer average calving interval might be associated with scarcity of feed and shortage of water for the long dry season of the year in the study area. The longer calving interval in younger cows might be due to higher nutrient requirement for growth in addition to milk production and maintenance thus delays the onset of postpartum heat. Similar effect of parity is reported by other scholars (Rege *et al.*, 1994; Addisu, 1999; Giday, 2001; Ababu, 2002; Getinet et al., 2009). However, others (Agyemang and Nkhonjera, 1990; Haile-Mariam and Mekonnen, 1996) reported non-significant effect of parity on CI. Brief information is summarized in the table below (table 1).

6

Table 1 Summary of age at first calving and calving interval (in month) of Ethiopian Indigenous breeds

Breeds	AFC	CI	References
Boran	57.6	13.8	Dejene (2014) for midland boran
	22.56	11.8	Meseret et al. (2014)
	42.8	14.9	Cited in Aynalem et al. (2011)
	57.6	20.7	Yifat et al. (2012)
	55.5	15.3	Solomon et al. (2011)
	58.8	16.8	Dejene (2014) for lowland boran
Fogera	51.4±0.05	21.18 ±0.70	Assemu et al. (2016)
	59.90+0.83	25.52+0.52	Damitie et al. (2015)
	52.4	19.3	Almaz (2012); Gebeyehu et al. (2005)
	53.4	17.5	Cited in Aynalem et al. (2011)
	63	37	Fasil et al. (2006)
	50.8+ 0.36		Menale et al. (2011)
Horro	58.08±0.07	21.08±0.3	Agere et al. (2012)
	53	17.6	Cited in Aynalem et al. (2011)
	50.0	12.2	Hailemariam and Mekonnen (1996)
	50	12	DADIS
Sheko	54.1	15.6	Takele et al.(2005)
		17.40± 0.20	Bayou et al.(2015)
Arsi	55.4±0.7		Chali (2014)
	3.39 years	14.2	Meseret et al. (2014)
	32.8	14.6	Mulugeta et al. (2008)
Barka	30.3	13.2	Million and Tadella(2003); Hailemariam and Mekonnen (1996)
Ogaden	49.2±4.43	16.43±0.44	Getinet et al.(2009)
	49.18±4.43		Getinet et al.(2005)
High land zebu	53	15.1	Niraj et al.(2014)
Metemma high land zebu	46.1	19.2	Tesfaye (2007)
Bagait	52.68±0.4	19.36±0.2	Tewelde et al.(2017)
	48.68±0.16	17.06±0.11	Mulugeta (2015)
	60	15.3	Cited in Aynalem et al. (2011)

Calving Interval (CI) and Age at First Calving (AFC) of Ethiopian Indigenous breeds

2.2.3. Number of services per-conception (NSPC):

Number of services per conception, which is defined as the number of services (natural or artificial) required for a successful conception, depends largely on the breeding system used, the reproductive health status of the animal, the management and feeding practices in a farm and the semen quality of AI or natural service bulls (Tewodros, 2008). Values of NSPC greater than 2 should be regarded as poor (Mukassa-Mugrewa, 1989). Number of service per conception is influenced by season; that is related to availability of feed, placenta expulsion time, lactation length and milk yield and parity (Hailemariam and Mekonnen, 1996; Gebeyehu *et al.*, 2005; Gebrekidan *et al.*, 2012).

NSPC obtained in this review for Boran breed was between 1.61 to 1.81 numbers, and that of Fogera was between 1.28±0.6 to 2±0.65 numbers. And that of Horro breed was 1.69 numbers. As I reviewed that the result obtained from Barka breed was shorter NSPC than any of others indigenous breed. This indicated that Barka breed can conceive better than others. The lower result for NSPC might be because of matting was conducted at the field where bulls and cows graze together naturally. Brief information is summarized in the table below (table 2).

2.2.4. Days open (DO):

Days open (also called calving-to-conception interval) is the period between calving and conception in cows (Tewodros, 2008). Days open is influenced by the length of time for the uterus to completely involutes, resumption of normal ovarian cycle, occurrence of silent ovulation, accuracy of heat detection, management, semen quality and skill of inseminator or efficiency of bull (Yosef, 2006; Melaku *et al.*, 2011). Days open affect lifetime production and generation intervals, and hence the annual genetic gain (Yosef, 2006). Getenet and Addisu (2006) and Ayenalem (2006) summarizes the reproductive performances of Fogera and Boran cattle, respectively in Ethiopia that was conducted by different authors in different years sourcing the data both at on-station and on-farm level. The authors summarize the performances of the respective breeds got decline from year to year and this decline, even in the same ranches, may be due to the deterioration of feed quality and invasion by unpalatable weeds of the grazing lands of the production sites; shrinkages of grazing land due to shift in farming system; lower level of selection of the best performing breeds. DO obtain in this review for Boran breed was between 141±7 to 339 days. DO obtain in this review for Fogera breed was between 285±4.3 to 298.4 days. DO obtain in this review for Horro breed was between 152 to 286.8±9 days. Cattles having shorter DO than any of others indigenous breed indicates that breed can have short calving to conception interval than others. Brief information is summarized in the table below (table 2).

2.2.5. Age at first service (AFS)

According to Giday (2001), age at first service (AFS) is the age at which heifers attain body condition and sexual maturity for accepting service for the first time. Age at first service signals the beginning of the heifer's reproduction and production and influences both the productive and reproductive life of the female through its effect on her life time calf crop. Age at first service is influenced by genotype, nutrition and other environmental factors (Zewdie, 2010). This reported an earlier age at puberty for F1 Friesian crosses than for indigenous zebu breeds. Age at first service was reported to be 42.24±0.05 to 44.8 months for Fogera breeds. In addition, age at first service reported in Ethiopia include about 32.4±1.4 to 53.9 months for Boran cattle and 48.42±0.05 to 55 months for Horro cattle. But the reviewed AFS result obtained for Ogaden breed was shorter than any of other indigenous breed. This indicated that Ogaden breed can have a short time requirement to attain body condition and sexual maturity than others. The desirable age at first calving in local breeds is 3 years. Prolonged age at first calving will have high production in the first lactation but the life time production will be decreased due to less no of calving. If the age at first calving is below optimum, the calves born are weak, difficulty in calving and less milk production in first lactation (Nerja and Kbrom, 2014). Brief information is summarized in the table below (table 2).

Table 2 Summary of age at first calving, days open and number of service per conception of Ethiopian Indigenous breeds

Breeds	AFS (month)	DO (days)	NSPC (no)	References
Boran	53.9	339	1.61	Yifat *et al.* (2012); Ababu, (2002)
	32.4 ± 1.4	141 ± 7	1.81	Haile *et al.* (2009b) 89. Haile-Mariam And Kassamersha (1994)
	42.7			Solomon *et al.* (2011)
Fogera	44.8	298.4	1.62	Almaz (2012); Gebeyehu *et al.*(2005); Giday (2001)
	42.24±0.05		1.54	Assemu *et al.* (2016); Gebeyehu *et al* (2004)
		285±4.3	1.28±0.6	Melaku *et al.* (2011)
			2±0.65	Tadele, A. and M. Nibret (2014)
Horro	48.42±0.05	286.8±9		Agere *et al.* (2012);
	50.72±0.6	152	1.69	Hailemariam and Mekonnen(1996)

	55			Zewdie wondatir, (2010)
Sheko	----------	248.32±6.02	-----------------	Bayou et al.(2015);
Arsi	41.8±08	211	2	Chali (2014); Mulugeta et al. (2008)
Barka	-------	253	1.11	Million and Tadella(2003); Hailemariam and Mekonnen (1996)
Ogaden	34.3±2.28	195	2	Getinet et al.(2009)
	34.4			Getinet et al.(2005)
Highland zebu	53	148	2.2	Niraj et al.(2014); Zewdie wondatir, (2010)
Metemma highland zebu	-------	204.1	1.74	Tesfaye (2007)
Bagait	43.97±0.3	229±36	----------	Tewelde et al.(2017); Teweldemedhn(2016)

Age at first service (AFS), Number of Service per Conception (NSPC) and Days Open (DO) of *Ethiopian Indigenous breeds*

2.3.*Growth performance* of indigenous Ethiopian cattle

Growth performance is very determinant parameter for beef and dual purpose cattle. It is primarily expressed and described by body weight and growth rate. Body weight changes of cattle are dependent on genetic and environmental factors. One of the major environmental factors that control cattle growth is feed to which the availability itself depends on climatic conditions. High growth rate is a very important parameter for beef enterprises. Mekonnen and Goshu (1996) reported that traits such as birth and weaning weight as well as growth and survival to weaning have important implications on herd productivity, management system, adaptability and breeding policy to be followed. Growth performance of an animal at various stages of the growth curve directly influences profitability in beef production systems (Newman and Coffey 1999). The expression of these traits is dependent on the animal's inherent growth ability and production environment (Davis 1993). These traits directly influence carcass (Pariacote et al. 1998), reproductive and milk production traits (Burrow 2001). They also form the basis of selection in many of the genetic improvement programs due to their early expression and ease of measurement.

2.3.1. Birth weight and weights at different ages

Birth weight was significantly affected by breed of calf and birth year; crossbred calves heavier than local breed calves and calves born in 2002 were heavier than those calves born in 2003. The effect of breed might be because of the heterosis effect (Demeke *et al.* 2003, Aynalem Haile, 2006). BWt obtained in this review for Boran (Demeke *et al.*2003), and Barka (Hailu D 2004) breeds were heavier than the values reported by other studies for Horro (Aynalem *et al.* 2011) ,Bagait (Aynalem *et al.* 2011), Fogera (Bitew *et al.* 2010),Ogaden (Getinet *et al.*2009), and Sheko (Bayou *et al.* 2015) breeds. As I reviewed that the result obtained from Sheko and Horro breed was shorter than any of others indigenous breed. This indicated that Sheko and Horro breed was born in small weight than others. This is because of that Short BWt was reported for growth performance of animal in the face of multiple stresses (nutrition, heat, parasites, disease and poor management), when small holder farmers are most vulnerable are the most important factors, resulting lower growth performance. Therefore manipulation of the management system could easily result in improved growth performance. Report by Kosgey (2004) indicated that improvement in performance can be achieved through improvement in management and feeding conditions and through genetic improvement by use of selecting genetically superior animals. Brief information is summarized in the table below (table 3).

Table 3 Birth weight and weight at different age of indigenous breed of Ethiopia

Breeds	BWT (kg)	WWT (kg)	ADG (g)/day	YWT (kg)	MWT (kg)	References
Boran	22.97	95.2	401.4	129.3	304	Aynalem *et al.* 2011; Demeke et al.2003
Fogera	22	92.9	319	125.2		Bitew *et al.* 2010; Giday 2003
Sheko	16.12 ± 0.22	76.29 ± 0.45	175.73±1.67	85.07 ± 0.50		Bayou *et al.* 2015
Horro	19.9	88	377.6	123	250	Aynalem *et al.* 2011; DAGRIS 2006 ; Demeke *et al.*2003
Barka	22.82± 0.93	99.01± 4.96	0.42±0.03kg	98	360	DAGRIS 2006; Hailu D 2004 Demeke *et al.*2003
Ogaden	21.50± 0.29	91.7±1 4.7	0.4±0.1k g	136.30±2.36	289.57	Getinet *et al.*2009; Getinet *et al.* 2005; Yesihak 2013
Bagait	22.6	92	385.3	124.5	380	Aynalem *et al.* 2011; Demeke *et al.*2003; DADIS

BWT-Birth weight; WWT-weaning weight; ADG- average daily gain; YWT-yearling weight; MWT-mature weight; SWT-slaughtering weight

2.3.2. Average daily body weight gain (ADG)

Average daily body weight gain from birth to one month was significantly affected by all fixed effects; crossbred calves, female calves, calves from the fourth parity dams, calves born in 2002 and calves born in the wet season had faster growth rate. Growth rates from birth to three and six months of age were influenced by breed and year of birth in that crossbred calves and calves born in 2002 had faster growth rate than their calves born in 2003 counterparts, respectively. The fixed effects considered for body weights affected weight gains similarly. Aynalem (2006) reported the effect of breed on daily gains of calves from birth to six months of age. Brief information is summarized in the table below (table 4) and above (table 3).

Table 4 Comparison between average body weight gain of boran and Kereyu Senga breeds with in different ages

Traits	Age groups								Sources
	2years of age		4years of age		6years of age		8years of age		
	Boran	Kereyu	Boran	Kereyu	Boran	Kereyu	Boran	Kereyu	
Average daily body weight gain (kg per day)	0.49±0.02	0.51 ± 0.03	0.63 ± 0.03	0.66 ± 0.03	0.65 ± 0.03	0.62 ± 0.04	0.65 ±0.03	0.6±0.05	Mohammed et al. 2008

The Boran breed with an estimated age of 6 and 8 years, gain averagely close to 0.65 kg per day. The Kereyu breed at the age groups of 4 year gain the highest average body weight from the other age groups of the same breed (0.66 kg) where as lower with increasing and decreasing ages. This is in agreement with the reports at Bako agricultural research center (unpublished) of 90-days experiment to examine the economical age at fattening Horro-Fresian crossbred bulls.

The results show that though older animals (37-48 months) ate more feeds and gained more weight than the younger (12-24 months). As indicated on the above table. This is in agreement with the reports of Tatek et al (2006 under publishing).

2.3.3. Carcass yield performance of indigenous Ethiopian cattle

Carcass traits describe the characteristics of beef. Broadly they are divided into carcass quality (composition) and carcass quantity traits. The carcass quality traits include: marbling score, fat thickness, kidney, pelvic and the heart fat percentages, rib eye area and yield grade. On the other hand, carcass quantity traits comprise of pre-slaughter live weight, hot carcass weight and dressing percentage (Pariacote et al. 1998). Carcass characteristics differ between breeds and are influenced by the plane of nutrition and production system (Keane and More O'Ferrall 1992). Selection for these traits is greatly influenced by the market demand. In the Ethiopian context, export markets demand lean meat whereas when the target is local market, fattened cattle are required regardless of animal's age. Therefore, the breeding, feeding and other management conditions should be designed in order to meet the demand of specific market (Haile A. et al 2008). The carcass characters for cattle have been studied mainly in regions where meat is valued in terms of quality (Wheeler et al. 2001).brief information is summarized in the table below.

Table 5 Literature of carcass characteristics of some Ethiopian beef cattle breeds

Carcass characteristics	Borena	Arsi
Slaughter weight	292	211
Empty body weight	261	189
Total carcass weight	147	103
Dressing%	50.2	48.3
Lean	92.8	72.8
Fat	16.7	12.6
Bone	30.8	21.5
Injesta	30.8	22.8
Internal organ	9	7.5
External organ	45.4	31.7
References	Nega T et al. 2002	Nega T et al. 2002

The effects of different compensatory growth on carcass characteristics of Boran and Arsi bulls are presented in Table 4. The interaction between feeding levels and breeds of animals were

13

consistently non-significant for carcass parameters measured except for internal organs (IO) and external organs (EO) slaughter weight (SLWT) and empty body weight (EBWT) were significantly different among treatments and breeds. Total carcass was also significantly different between breeds. Dressing percentage, fat, lean and bone yield were significantly different among treatments and between breeds. Although the Boran and Arsi bulls were at the same age at the commencement of the study, the preparation of lean and bone of the Boran was 27.7% and 43.2%, respectively, which was higher than the Arsi. The quantity of Injesta was significantly affected by breed but the difference among treatments was not significant. Internal organs were not significantly affected by treatments but affected by breeds. External organs had also similar trend with the live weight of animals at slaughter and total carcass. The overall carcass characteristics indicated declining trends with increasing levels of feed restriction. This may be because of different levels of feed restriction.

Table 6 Carcass yield performance of the two Ethiopian indigenous cattle breed

Parameters	Breeds		
	Kereyu	Boran	References
Hot carcass, kg	106.29 ± 9.96b	128.08 ± 11.89a	
Dressing percentage	44.93 1.16 a	47.49 ± 2.08 a	
Pelvic fat, g	266.65 ±103.56b	559.09 ± 90.43a	
Scrotal fat, kg	0.77 ± 0.12b	1.26 ± 0.17a	Mohammed et al.
Heart fat, g	135.85 ± 54.66a	507.54 ± 218.19a	2008
Kidney fat, kg	0.98 ± 0.15b	1.66 ± 0.22a	
Fat thickness, mm	3.25 ± 0.55a	4.25 ±0.71a	
Rib eye area	173.50 ± 12.50b	223.17 ± 14.70a	

Similarly to that of average body weight gain, hot carcass and rib eye area were recorded higher in Boran breed than Kereyu breed. Fat thickness and dressing percentage of Boran breed higher than Kereyu breed, even though not statistically significant. This is in agreement with the reports of Tesfaye Lemma *et al* (2007) on the effect of four different basal diets on the carcass composition of finishing Boran bulls, There was no significant difference in heart and Omental and mesenteric fat weights, and back fat thickness among rations.

At the chilling floor, left side of each carcass were sawed at the 12th and 13th ribs to measure the rib eye area and fat thickness of the longissimus muscle. Rib eye area was measured by placing grid plastic paper (Iowa State University extension and outreach) on the cut surface of the rib eye and counting all squares in which lean surrounds a dot as per the guidance described by manufacturer of the plastic grid. The number of squares counted was divided by 10. The resulting number was the area of the rib eye in square inches USDA (1996). Fat thickness was measured by ruler graduated in millimeters. The dressing percentage was evaluated according to Warriss, P.D. (2000). Dressing Percentage (DP) was calculated as:

Dressing Percentage = Hot Carcass Weight/ Live weight×100

As mentioned in the above main title effect of age and breeds of cattle on carcass and meat characteristics is summarized as follows in table form.

Table 7 Effects of cattle of age and breed on carcass characteristics.

Parameters	Age (year)	Breeds			References
		Arsi	Boran	Harar	
Live	4-6	167.33±14.64	200.2±9.65	181±18.95	
weight(kg)	7-9	192±9.17	433±39.27	155.75±43.84	T. D. Tefera et
	<3	69.6±8.02	57.2±9.26	85±19.76	al.(2019)
Carcass	4-6	72.83±16.51	92.47±7.21	86.8±12.56	
weight (kg)	7-9	87.67±5.13	209.73±11.5	72±25.32	
	<3	51.6±5.42	41.8±1.3	46.4±1.2	
Dressing	4-6	44.31±13.6	46.17±2.43	47.8±1.93	
percentage	7-9	45±6.9	48.63±3.59	45.64±4.4	
(%)	<3	16.56±2.88	11.79±5.2	15.62±2.31	
Forequarter	4-6	19.24±5.76	33.55±22.76	21.47±2.83	
(kg)	7-9	22.69±0.88	56.42±4.6	28.45±1.44	
	<3	16.77±2.35	14.04±2.73	15.64±1.99	T. D. Tefera et
Hindquarter	4-6	16.55±2.94	22.12±3.51	21.21±23.85	al.(2019)
(kg)	7-9	18.26±0.21	45.34±4.23	23.83±2.1	
	<3	7.28±0.5	4.78±0.86	6.06±1.63	
Rib Eye Area	4-6	7.53±0.93	7.38±1.24	6.84±1.08	
(SI)	7-9	7.83±1.27	10.25±1.16	7.98±1.28	

Breed and age of cattle had significant influence on live and carcass weights, forequarter and hindquarter weights, and rib eye area (Table 6). Boran between 7 and 9 years of age were higher both in live and carcass weights than Arsi and Harar cattle breeds. The higher live and carcass weights of Boran breed compared to other breeds in the country were similarly reported by Yesihak, M.Y. (2015). Higher Boran live and carcass weight might be due to the improvement program practiced for the breed since 1960 Aynalem H et al. (2011). The difference in live and carcass weight of Boran breed over Arsi and Harar cattle breed might be also due to the feeding system on which these breeds were finished, i.e. the Boran was finished in ranch condition while the Arsi and Harar under smallholder feeding regime with grazing and crop residues as a major feed resource. Wheat, barley straw, and maize/sorghum Stover were the major sources of crop residues used as feed in the latter breeds as they were managed in mixed crop livestock system. Mean carcass weight of Boran breed between 7 to 9 years in the present review was higher than the average carcass weight of 154 kg reported by Yesihak, M.Y. (2015) for the same breed slaughtered at export abattoir in Ethiopia. The carcass weights of Arsi and Harar cattle breeds were lower than the carcass weight of cattle (135 kg) slaughtered at local abattoirs in Ethiopia Yesihak, M.Y. and Webb, E.C. (2014).

The dressing percentage of Boran breed in the present study was lower than that reported for the same breed reported by Yesihak, M.Y. (2015) and Aynalem H et al. (2011) and for Ogaden cattle Yoseph, M et al. (2011), which was 56%. Dressing percentage for Arsi and Harar cattle breeds were comparable with the same parameter reported for cattle slaughtered at local and export abattoirs in Ethiopia, which was 46.78% Yesihak, M.Y. (2015). Moreover, the dressing percentage in the present review was comparable to Simmental bulls, Brazil Nellore breed and their crossbred bulls Ustuner, H. et al.(2017), Rotta, P.P.et al. (2009), Zawadzki, F.et al. (2011), Cruz, O.T.B.et al. (2014), Barcellos, V.C.et al.(2017).

Despite the significant difference in live and carcass weight, age didn't also influenced dressing percentage. This may be due to similar proportions of carcass to live weight ratio across different age groups since carcass dressing percentage is related to body weight Macedo, L.M.et al (2008), Pogorzelska-Przybyłek, P.et al.(2018). Forequarter mean weight of Boran in age category of 4 - 6 years was higher than Arsi and Harar. At 7 - 9 years, mean of Forequarter of Boran was higher than Arsi and Harar. The result of this study was comparable with the finding of Yesihak, M.Y. (2015) on local Ethiopian cattle breeds that showed mean forequarter of Boran at 4 - 6 years similar with Barka (34.28 kg), and Harar at 7 - 9 years with Raya (29.78 kg) breeds. The hindquarter weight of Arsi breed in age categories from 4 - 6 years was relatively lower than their counter part Boran and Harar breeds.

Rib eye area is an objective assessment of muscling and an indicator of total muscle in the carcass or live animal Greiner, S.P. (2002); Greenfield, J.B. (2009). It is an indicator trait of carcass composition associated with muscularity and yield of high value-added cuts Baldassini, W.A.et al. (2017), Aranha, A.S.et al. (2018). At 7 - 9 years of age, Boran breed recorded significantly higher

16

value in mean rib eye area than Arsi and Harar while all cattle breeds (4 - 6 years) had similar rib eye area. In all cattle breed rib eye area showed increasing trend across the age category. The trend of rib eye area content in Boran was higher than Arsi and Harar. This implies that Boran carcass has a large proportion of lean muscle.

3. CONCLUSION AND RECOMMENDATION

Generally, the reproductive and productive performance of Boran, Fogera, Ogaden, Barca, and Arsi cattle are relatively better than the values reported for most other tropical and particularly Ethiopian cattle breeds. However it is declining through time which implies the breed influenced by environmental factors or poor management as the result of several researchers indicate in the range of timeframe. Therefore strategic improvement of feeding, breeding, management and follow up is important to boost up the reproductive and productive performance as well as genetic maintenance of the breed. From the above reviews the following recommendation were forwarded:

❖ Indigenous beef cattle breeds had the ability of better adaptability of environments; there should be a controlled crossbreeding and selection strategy in line with conservation of the local adaptive traits of the breeds.

❖ Training and awareness creation should be given particularly to the farmers to increase the productive and reproductive performance of the beef cattle and livelihood of the farmers through improved management practices.

❖ In Ethiopia, genetic improvement of the indigenous cattle for dairy production, focusing on crossbreeding, has been practiced for the last five decades, albeit with little success. Selection as an improvement tool has been given less emphasis and as such there have been no systematic and organized selection schemes for cattle genetic improvement in Ethiopia. In addition, little or no genetic improvement work targeted at improving beef production has been undertaken so far. Therefore, there is a need to develop effective and sustainable genetic improvement schemes for indigenous cattle breeds of Ethiopia.

❖ The significant effects of season of calving on the performance of traits suggested that improvement in feed and management is the key factor for further improvement of these local breeds. In order to improve the relatively the poor milk yield, the extended AFC and CI, as well as the short LL, improving the feeding system, providing better health management, genetic improvement of local bred through crossbreeding are necessary so as to further exploit the optimum level of reproductive and productive performance of indigenous cattle.

❖ Ethiopian Boran breed can be used for beef or dairy production. Literature reports and my own review indicate that growth and reproductive performance of the breed are fairly good

18

compared to some indigenous breeds and this attributes make Boran cattle good beef animal. The milk production potential of Ethiopian Boran has not been improved. However, if concerted efforts can be made in terms of improving the potential of the breed and the whole horizon of the value chain can be worked on, the breed can substantially contribute to the Ethiopia's economic development and wellbeing of its people.

❖ Kereyu breed at younger age and in good management perform more body weight gain than the known Borana breed bulls. However, in carcass yield aspect and at older age daily body weight gain, Borana breed perform better than Kereyu breed outside of their native habitat. The study in general indicated that the grazing performance of the Kereyu breed is lower than the Borana breeds. Kereyu breed needs more investigation to see their potentials in all aspects.

❖ From the review, it was concluded that age and breeds of cattle had significantly influence on carcass and meat characteristics. In old age (7 - 9 years) Boran better performed than Arsi and Harar in live weight, carcass weight, forequarter, rib eye area, heart and ommental fat, rib cut percentage, chuck cuts weight and loin weight. Arsi bulls yielded higher meat yield percent at an early age (<3 years), while decreasing as the age advanced and the meat yield percentage from Harar cattle increased linearly as the age advanced up to 9 years. Live and hot carcass weight, chuck, sirloin and tenderloin could be reliable measurement in estimation of meat yield. Therefore, to determine whether variations were due to genetic or environmental cause's evaluation of the three breeds under similar feeding was recommended.

REFERENCES

Ababu D (2002). Evaluation of performance of Boran cows in the production of crossbred dairy heifers at Abernosa ranch Ethiopia. MSc Thesis. Alemaya, Ethiopia.

Addisu, B. 1999. Evaluation of reproductive and growth performance of Fogera cattle and their F1 Friesian crosses at Metekel Ranch, Ethiopia. MSc Thesis Alemaya University, Alemaya, Ethiopia.

Addisu, B., T. Mengistie, K. Adebabay, M. Getinet T. Asaminew, M. Tezera and G. Gebeyehu (2010). Milk yield and calf growth performance of cattle under partial suckling system at Andassa Livestock Research Centre, North West Ethiopia. Livestock Research for Rural Development. http://www.lrrd.org/lrrd22/8/bite22136.htm

Agere M, Aynalem H, Tadelle D, Yoseph M (2012). On farm characterization of Horro cattle breed production systems in western Oromia, Ethiopia. Livest. Res. Rural Dev. 24(6):100.

Almaz B. (2012). Genetic parameter estimation of growth and reproduction traits of Fogera cattle at Metekel ranch, Amhara region, Ethiopia. MSc thesis submitted to Bahir Dar University college of Agriculture and Environmental science, Bahir Dar, Ethiopia.

Aranha, A.S., Andrighetto, C., Lupatini, G.C., Mateus, G.P., Ducatti, C.R., Roça, O., Martins, M.B., Santos, J.A.A., Luz, P.A.C., Utsunomiya, A.T.H. and Athayde, N.B. (2018) Performance, Carcass, and Meat Characteristics of Two Cattle Categories Finished On Pasture during the Dry Season with Supplementation in Different Forage Allowance. Arquivo Brasileiro de Medicina Veterinária e Zootecnia , 70, 517-524. https://doi.org/10.1590/1678-4162-9576

Assemu T, Dilip K, Solomon, Getinet M (2017). Conservation and Improvement Strategy for Fogera Cattle: A Lesson for Ethiopia Indigenous Cattle Breed Resource Hindawi. Adv. Agric. 2017, Article ID 2149452, 12p.

Ayalew W, King J, Bruns E, Rischkowsky B (2003). Economic evaluation of smallholder subsistence livestock production: lessons from an Ethiopian goat development program. Ecol. Econ. 45(3): 473–485.

Aynalem H, Workneh A, Noah K, Tadelle D, Azage T (2011). Breeding strategy to improve Ethiopian Boran cattle for meat and milk production. IPMS (Improving Productivity and Market Success) of Ethiopian Farmers Project Working Paper 26. Nairobi, Kenya, ILRI.

Baldassini, W.A., Cahdulo, L.A.L., Silva, J.A.V., et al . (2017) Meat Quality Traits of Nellore Bulls According to Different Degrees of Backfat Thickness: A Multivariate Approach. Animal Production Science , 57, 363-370. https://doi.org/10.1071/AN15120

Barcellos, V.C., Mottin, C., Passetti, R.A.C., Guerrero, A., Carlos Emanuel Eiras, C.E., Prohman, P.E., Vital, A.C.P. and Ivanor Nunes do Prado, I.N. (2017) Carcass Characteristics and Sensorial Evaluation of Meat from Nellore Steers and Crossbred Angus vs. Nellore Bulls. Animal Science Journal , 39, 437-448. https://doi.org/10.4025/actascianimsci.v39i4.36692

Bayou E, Haile A, Gizaw S, Mekasha Y (2015). Evaluation of non-genetic factors affecting calf growth, reproductive performance and milk yield of traditionally managed Sheko cattle in southwest Ethiopia. SpringerPlus 4:568.

Belay D, Yisehak K and Janssens GP (2012). Productive and Reproductive Performance of Zebu X Holstein-Friesian Crossbred Dairy Cows in Jimma Town, Oromia, Ethiopia. Global Veterinarian 8 (1): 67-72.

Belete A, 2006. Studies on cattle milk and meat production in Fogera woreda: production systems, constraints and opportunities for development. Debub university, Awassa, Ethiopia.

Burrow, H.M. 2001. Variances and covariances between productive and adaptive traits and temperament in a composite breed of tropical beef cattle. Livestock Production Science. 70:213-233.

Central Statistical Agency (CSA) (2009). Agricultural sample survey (2008/2009). Report on livestock and livestock characteristics. Statistical bulletin 446. Addis Ababa, Ethiopia.

Central Statistical Agency (CSA) (2010/2011). Federal Democratic Republic of Ethiopia: Central statistical agency; Agricultural sample survey 2010/11 [2003 E.C.], volume 2: Report on livestock and livestock characteristics (private peasant holdings), Statistical bulletin 505, February 2011, Addis Ababa, Ethiopia

Central Statistical Agency (CSA) (2014/2015). Federal democratic republic of Ethiopia: Agricultural sample survey, 2014/2015 (2007 E.C.) (September – January 2014/2015), volume-2: Report on crop and livestock product utilization (private peasant holdings, Meher season), statistical bulletin-578, June, 2015, Addis Ababa, Ethiopia.

Central Statistical Agency (CSA) (2015/2016). Federal democratic republic of Ethiopia: Key findings of the 2015/2016 (2008 E.C) agricultural sample surveys: Country summary, July, 2016, Addis Ababa, Ethiopia.

Central Statistical Agency (CSA) (2016/2017). Federal democratic republic of Ethiopia: Agricultural sample survey 2016/17 [2009 E.C.], volume-2: Report on livestock and livestock characteristics (private peasant holdings). Statistical bulletin-585, April 2017, Addis Ababa, Ethiopia.

Cruz, O.T.B., Valero, M.V., Zawadzki, F., Rivaroli, D.C., Prado, R.M., Lima, B.S. and Prado, I.N. (2014) Effect of Glycerine and Essential Oils (Anacardium occide ntale and Ricinus communis) on Animal Performance, Feed Efficiency and Carcass Characteristics of Crossbred Bulls Finished in a Feedlot System. Italian Journal of Animal Science , 13, 790-797. https://doi.org/10.4081/ijas.2014.3492

DAGRIS (Domestic Animal Genetic Resources Information System) (2004) International Livestock Research Institute. Addis Ababa, Ethiopia. http://wwwdagris.ilri.cgiar.org. Accessed 5 Feb 2013

DAGRIS (Domestic Animal Genetic Resources Information System). 2006. (eds. Rege JEO, Ayalew W, Getahun E, Hanotte O and Dessie T). International Livestock Research Institute, Addis Ababa, Ethiopia. http://dagris.ilri.cgiar.org.

Damitie K, Kefyalew A, Endalkachew G (2015). Reproductive and Productive Performance of Fogera Cattle in Lake Tana Watershed, North Western Amhara, Ethiopia. J. Reprod. Infertil. 6(2):56-62.

Davis, G.P (1993). Genetic parameters for tropical beef cattle in Northern Australia: A review. Australian Journal of Agricultural Research. 44:179-198.

Dejene T (2014). Assessment of dairy cattle husbandry and breeding management practices of lowland and mid-highland agro-ecologies of Borana zone. Anim. Vet. Sci. 2(3):62-69.

Demeke, S., Neser, F.W.C. and Schoeman, S.J. 2003. Early growth performance of Bos Taurus × Bos indicus cattle crosses in Ethiopia: Evaluation of different crossbreeding models. J. Anim.Breed. Genet. 120:39-50.

Demeke, S., Neser, F.W.C. and Schoeman, S.J. 2004b. Estimates of genetic parameters for Boran, Friesian, and crosses of Friesian and Jersey with the Boran cattle in the tropical highlands of Ethiopia: milk production traits and cow weight. J. Anim. Breed. Genet. 121:163-175.

22

Demissu Hundie, Fekadu Beyene, and Gemeda Duguma (2013). Early Growth and Reproductive Performances of Horro Cattle and their F1 Jersey Crosses in and around Horro-Guduru Livestock Production and Research Center, Ethiopia. ISSN: 2226-7522(Print) and 2305-3327 (Online).

Domestic Animal Diversity Information System (DADIS). (Access date: 20/11/2017) at http://dad.fao.org/, Number of breeds by species and country.

Domestic Animal Genetic Resources Information System (DAGRIS) (2007). Domestic Animal Genetic Resources Information System (DAGRIS). (eds. S. Kemp, Y. Mamo, B. Asrat and T. Dessie). International Livestock Research Institute, Addis Ababa, Ethiopia.

Domestic Animal Genetic Resources Information System (DAGRIS) (Access date: 21/11/2017) at http://www.dagris.info/countries/192/breeds, Livestock breeds in Ethiopia.

EARO, 1999, Livestock research strategy (unpublished), Addis Ababa, Ethiopia.

Estefanos T, Tesfaye A, Feyisa H, Gashaye W, Tatek W, Tesfaye K and Osho T, 2014. Traditional cattle production in the highlands of Hararge: Case study for East and West Zones of the high lands of Harerge, Eastern Ethiopia. Basic Research Journal of Agricultural Science and Review ISSN 23156880 Vol. 3(12) pp. 122-130 December 2014.

Ethiopian Institute of Biodiversity Conservation (EIBC) (2004). The State of Ethiopia's Farm Animal Genetic Resources: Country Report. A Contribution to the First Report on the State of the World's Animal Genetic Resources. IBC. May 2004. Addis Ababa, Ethiopia.

Ethiopian Institute of Biodiversity Conservation (EIBC) (2012c). Ethiopia's Strategy and Plan of Action for Conservation, Sustainable use and Development of Animal Genetic Resources, Addis Ababa, Ethiopia.

FAO (Food and Agriculture Organization) (1993). Livestock and improvements of pasture, feed and forage. Committee on Agriculture, 12th session, item 7, 26 April–4 May 1993. FAO, Rome, Italy.

Fasil G, Workneh A (2006). On-farm phenotypic characterization of indigenous cattle populations of Awi, East and West Gojjam Zones of Amhara Region, Ethiopia. Res. J. Agric. Environ. Manage. 3(4):227-237.

Firew, T. (2007): Evaluation of alternative feed resources for ruminants under arid zones of the tropics and subtropics: the case of cactus pear (Oppuntia ficus-indica) in Ethiopia. Ph.D. Thesis. Humboldt University of Berlin, Germany.

Food and Agriculture Organization (FAO) (2005). Rome, Italy.

Food and Agriculture Organization (FAO) (2009). Contributions of Smallholder Farmers and Pastoralists to the Development, use, and Conservation of Animal Genetic Resources. Commission on Genetic Resources for food and Agriculture. Intergovernmental Technical Working Group on Animal Genetic Resources for Food and Agriculture. 5th Session, Rome, 28-30 January 2009. 40 p.

Gebeyehu G, Asmare A, Asseged B (2005). Reproductive performances of Fogera cattle and their Friesian crosses in Andassa ranch, Northwestern Ethiopia. Available at: http://www.lrrd.org/lrrd17/12/gosh17131.htm.

Gebrekidan T.W, Zeleke M.Z and Gangwar, S.K (2012). Reproductive and productive performance of dairy Cattle in central zone of Tigray, northern Ethiopia.

Getinet M, Hegde B and Workneh A (2005). On Station Ex-Situ Phenotypic and Morphological Characterization of Ogaden Cattle at Alemaya University, Ethiopia. MSc Thesis Abstracts, School of Animal and Range Sciences of Alemaya University, Volume I (19802013).

Getinet M, Workneh A and Hegde BP (2009). Growth and Reproductive performance of Ogaden cattle at Haramaya University, Ethiopia. Ethiop. J. Anim. Prod. 9(1):1607-3835.

Giday, Y.E., 2001. Assessment of calf crop productivity and total herd life of Fogera cows at Andassa ranch in North-western Ethiopia. MSc Thesis, Alemaya University, Alemaya, Ethiopia.

Greenfield, J.B. (2009) Carcass Trends in Beef Cattle Shown at the Clarksville Better Beef Show.

Greiner, S.P. (2002) Understanding Expected Progeny Differences (EPDs). Publication Number 400-804. Virginia Tech University: Virginia Cooperative Extension, College Town

Habtamu L, Kelay B, Desie S (2010). Study on the reproductive performance of Jersey cows at Wolaita Sodo dairy farm, Southern Ethiopia. Ethiop. Vet. J. 14(1):53-70.

Haile, A., Joshi, B.K., Workneh Ayalew, Azage Tegegne, Singh A. and Zelalem Yilma. 2008. Genetic evaluation of Boran cattle and their crosses with Holstein Friesian in central Ethiopia: milk composition traits. Journal of Cell and Animal Biology. 2(10):171-176.

Haile-Mariam M. and Kassa-Mersha H (1994). Genetic and environmental effects on age at first calving and calving interval of naturally bred Boran (zebu) cows in Ethiopia. Animal Production, 58: 329-334.

Hailemariam M, Mekonnen, G (1996). Reproductive performance of Zebu, Friesian and Friesian. Zebu crosses. Trop. Agric. 73:142-147.

Haile-Mariam, M. And H. Kassamersha, 1994. Genetic and environmental effects on age at first calving and calving interval of naturally bred Boran (zebu) cows in Ethiopia. Animal Production, 58: 329-334.

Keane, M.G. and More O'Ferrall, G.J. 1992. Comparison of Friesian, Canadian Hereford × Friesian and Simmental × Friesian steers for growth and carcass composition. Animal Production. 55:377-387.

Kelay B.D (2002). Analyses of Dairy Cattle Breeding Practices in Selected Areas of Ethiopia. Dissertation. http://edoc.hu-berlin.de/dissertationen/desta-kelay-belihu-2.

Kosgey IS (2004) Breeding objectives and breeding strategies for small ruminant in the tropics. (unpublished PhD thesis, University of Wageningen).

Macedo, L.M., Prado, I.M., Prado, J.M., Rotta, P., Prado, R.M., Souza, N.E. and Prado, I.N. (2008) Chemical Composition and Fatty Acids Profile of Five Carcass Cuts of Crossbred Heifers Finished in Feedlot. Semina : Ciências Agrárias , 29, 597-608.

Mekonnen Haile-Mariam and Goshu Mekonnen. 1996. Reproductive performance of Fogera cattle and their Friesian crosses. Eth. J. Agric. Sci. 9(2):95-114.

Melaku, M., M. Zeleke, M. Getinet and T. Mengistie 2011. Reproductive performances of Fogera cattle at Metekel Cattle breeding and multiplication Ranch, North West Ethiopia. J. Anim. Feed Res., 1: 99-106.

Melku M, Kefyalew A, and Solomon G, (2016). Milk Production and Reproductive Performance of Local and Crossbreed Dairy Cows in Selected Districts of West Gojam Zone, Amhara Region, Ethiopia, MSc thesis, Bahir Dar, Ethiopia.

Menale M, Mekuriaw Z, Mekuriaw G, Taye M (2011). Reproductive performance of Fogera cattle at Metekel Cattle Breeding and Multiplication Ranch, North West Ethiopia. J. Anim. Feed Res. 1(3):99-106.

Meseret T, Berihu G and Berihun A (2014). Survey on Reproductive Performance of Smallholder Dairy Cows in Hawassa City, Ethiopia. J. Reprod. Infertil. 5(3):69-75.

Million T, Tadelle D (2003). Milk production performance of Zebu, Holstein Friesian and their crosses in Ethiopia. Livest. Res. Rural Dev. (15)3:1-9.

Ministry of Agriculture and Rural Development (MoARD) (2007). Livestock Development Master Plan Study, Phase I Report – Data Collection and Analysis, Volume B – Meat Production.

MOA (Ministry of Agriculture), Animal and fishery resources development main department, Fattening extension manual, FLDP, 1996, Addis Ababa, Ethiopia, 83 pp.

Mohammed N, Tesfaye L, Takele F, Hailu D, Tatek W, Tesfaye A and Birhanu S(2008). Comparison of body weight gain performance and carcass characteristics of the two Ethiopian cattle breeds under natural pasture grazing management in Livestock Research for Rural Development 20(8):#117 *with* 169 Reads Adami Tulu Agricultural research center, Ziway, Ethiopia.

Mostert B.E., van der Westhuizen R.R. and Theron H.E (2010). Calving interval genetic parameters and trends for dairy breeds in South Africa. South African Journal of Animal Science 2010, 40 (2).

Mukasa-Mugerwa E (1989). A review of reproductive performance of female Bos indicus Zebu cattle. ILCA Monograph 6. Addis Ababa, Ethiopia. pp151.

Mukassa- Mugerwa, E. and Azage, T (1991). Reproductive Performance in Ethiopian Zebu (Bos indicus) Cattle: Constraints and impact on production. An invited paper presented at Fourth National livestock Improvement Conference, Addis Ababa, Ethiopia, 13-15 Nov. 1991. Inustitute of Agricultural Research (IAR) Pp 16-18.

Mulugeta A and Belayeneh A (2013). Reproductive and lactation performances of dairy cows in Chacha Town and nearby selected kebeles, North Shoa Zone, Amhara Region, Ethiopia, World Journal of Agricultural Sciences ,1(1), pp. 008017.Available online at http://wsrjournals.org/journal/wjas ISSN 2329-9312 ©2013 World Science Research Journals.

Mulugeta A, Azage T, Hegde BP (2008). Reproductive performance of dairy cows in the Yerer Watershed, Oromiya Region, Ethiopia. Proceedings of the 16th annual conference of the Ethiopian Society of Animal Production (ESAP) held in Addis Ababa, Ethiopia. Part II: Technical Session. pp. 219-229.

Mulugeta A, Azage T, Hegde BP (2008). Reproductive performance of dairy cows in the Yerer Watershed, Oromiya Region, Ethiopia. Proceedings of the 16th annual conference of the

Ethiopian Society of Animal Production (ESAP) held in Addis Ababa, Ethiopia. Part II: Technical Session. pp. 219-229

Mulugeta Ayalew, Azage Tegegne, and B.P. Hegde (2008). Reproductive performance of dairy cows in the Yerer Watershed, Oromiya Region, Ethiopia. Proceedings of the 16th annual conference of the Ethiopian Society of Animal Production (ESAP) held in Addis Ababa, Ethiopia. Part II: Technical Session, 219-229pp.

Mulugeta FG (2015). Production system and phenotypic characterization of Begait cattle and effects of supplementation with concentrate feeds on milk yield and composition of Begait cows in Humera ranch, western Tigray, Ethiopia. PhD Dissertation, Addis Ababa University, College of Veterinary Medicine and Agriculture, Debre Zeit, Ethiopia.

Nega Tolla, Tadele Mirkena and Asfaw Yimegnuhal. 2002 Comparision of the efficiency of compensatory growth of Borana and Arsi cattle in Ethiopia. Ethiopian Journal of Animal Production 2 (1):11-23.

Negassa, S., Rashid, S., Gebremedhin, B. (2011). Livestock Production and Marketing. Development Strategy and Governance Division, International Food Policy Research Institute, Ethiopia Strategy Support Program II (ESSP II), ESSP II Working Paper 26, Ethiopia.

Newman, S. and Coffey, S.G. 1999. Genetic Aspects of Cattle Adaptation in the Tropics. CAB Publications.

Nibret M and Tadele A (2014). Study on Reproductive Performance of Indigenous Dairy Cows at Small Holder Farm Conditions in and Around Maksegnit Town, Global Veterinarian 13 (4): 450-454, 2014.

Niraj K, Kbrom T and Abraha B, (2014). Reproductive performance of dairy cows under farmer's management in and around Mekelle, Ethiopia, College of Veterinary Medicine, Mekelle University, P.O.Box-231, nirajjha1925@yahoo.com of Amhara region. 4th ed. Bahir Dar, Ethiopia.

Niraj K, Yemane A, Berihu G, Yohannes HW (2014). Productive and Reproductive Performance of Local Cows under Farmer's Management in and around Mekelle, Ethiopia. IOSR J. Agric. Vet. Sci. 7(5):21-24.

Nuraddis I, Ashebir A and Shiferaw M (2011). Assessment of reproductive performance of crossbred dairy cattle (Holstein Friesian X zebu) in Gondar town. Global Veterinaia 6(6): 561-566. IDOSI Publications, 2011. http://idosi.org/gv/GV6(6)11/12.pdf.

Olawumi S.O. and Salako A.E (2010). Genetic Parameters and Factors Affecting Reproductive Performance of White Fulani Cattle in Southwestern, Nigeria. Global Veterinaria 5 (5): 255-258, 2010.

Pariacote, F., Van Vleck, L.D. and Hunsley, R.E. 1998. Genetic and phenotypic parameters for carcass traits of American Shorthorn beef cattle. Journal of Animal Science. 76:2584-2588.

Pogorzelska-Przybyłek, P., Nogalski, Z., Sobczuk-Szul, M., Purwin, G. and Kubiak, D. (2018) Carcass Characteristics and Meat Quality of Holstein-Friesian × Hereford Cattle of Different Sex Categories and Slaughter Ages. Archives Animal Breeding , 61, 253-261. https://doi.org/10.5194/aab-61-253-2018

Prabhakar and Addisu (2004). Reproductive and growth performance of Fogera cattle and their F1 Friesian crosses at Metekel ranch, Ethiopia. AGRIS: International Information System for the Agricultural science and technology.

Pryce, J. E., Royal, M. D., Garnsorthy P. C. and Mao, I. L (2004). Fertility in the high producing dairy cow. Livestock Prod. Sci., 86: 125.135.

Rege JED (1999) The state of African cattle genetic resources I. Classification framework and identification of threatened and extinct breeds. Anim Genetic Res Inform 25:1–25

Rege JEO, Aboagye GS, Ahah S and Ahunu BK (1994). Crossbreeding Jersey with Ghana Short horn and Sokoto Gudali cattle in a tropical environment: additive and heterotic effects for milk production, reproduction and calf growth traits. Animal Production 59: 21-29.

Rotta, P.P., Prado, R.M., Prado, I.N., Valero, M.V., Visentainer, J.V. and Silva, R.R. (2009) The Effects of Genetic Groups, Nutrition, Finishing Systems and Gender of Brazilian Cattle on Carcass Characteristics and Beef Composition and Appearance: A Review. Asian Australasian Journal of Animal Sciences, 22, 1718-1734. https://doi.org/10.5713/ajas.2009.90071

Shawel Betru and H Kawashima Livestock Research for Rural Development 21 (9) 2009">Livestock Research for Rural Development 21 (9) 2009 Pattern and determinants of meat consumption in urban and rural Ethiopia.

Shiferaw G, Hegde BP, Workneh A (2006). In-Situ Phenotypic Characterization of Kereyu Cattle Type in Fentalle District of Oromia Region, Ethiopia. MSc Thesis Abstracts, School of Animal and Range Sciences of Alemaya University, Volume I (1980-2013).

Shiferaw Garoma Asella School of Agriculture, Adama Science and Technology University, P.O.Box 193, Ethiopia. Accepted 30 January, 2014

Solomon T, Tadelle D, Kefelegn K (2011). On-Farm Phenotypic Characterization of Boran Cattle Breed in Dire District of Borana Zone, Oromia Region, Ethiopia. MSc Thesis Abstracts, School of Animal and Range Sciences of Alemaya University, Volume I (19802013).

Tadele, A. and M. Nibret, 2014. Study on reproductive performance of indigenous dairy cows at small holder farmers condition in and around Makisegnit Town. Global Veterinaria, 13: 450-454

Takele T, Workneh A, Hegde BP (2005). On-Farm Phenotypic Characterization of Sheko Breed of Cattle and their Habitat in Bench Maji Zone, Ethiopia. MSc Thesis Abstracts, School of Animal and Range Sciences of Alemaya University, Volume I (1980-2013).

Tefera, T.D., Mummed, Y.Y., Kurtu, M.Y., Letta, M.U., O'Quine, T.G. and Vipham, J.L. (2019) Effect of Age and Breeds of Cattle on Carcass and Meat Characteristics of Arsi, Boran, and Harar Cattle in Ethiopia. Open Journal of Animal Sciences,9,367-383. https://doi.org/10.4236/ojas.2019.93030

Tesfaye Lemma, Tesfa Geleta, Amsalu Sisay and Tekele Abebe 2007 Effects of four different basal diets on the carcass composition of finishing Borana bulls. Journal of Cell and Animalbiology1(2):1518http://www.academicjournals.org/jcab/PDF/Pdf2007/Sept/Lemma%20et%20al.pdf.

Tesfaye M (2007). Characterization of cattle milk and meat production, processing and marketing system in Metema district, Ethiopia. MSc. Thesis; Hawassa University.

Tewelde G, Sintayehu Y, Sandip B (2017). Some morphometric, production and reproduction traits of Begait cattle reared in Tigray region of Ethiopia. Wayamba J. Anim. Sci. – ISSN: 2012-578X; P1571 - P1585, 2017, First Submitted June 08, 2017; Number 1498735834.

Teweldemedhn M (2016). Characterization of Production System, Productive and Reproductive Performance and Morphological Traits of Begait Cattle in Western Zone of Tigray Region, Ethiopia. MSc Thesis, Haramaya University, Ethiopia.

Tewodros Bimerew (2008). Assessment of Productive and Reproductive Performance of Indigenous and Crossbred Cattle under Smallholder Management System in North Gondar, Amhara Region. MSc. Thesis; Mekelle University, Ethiopia.

USDA United States Department of Agriculture (1996) Standards for Grades of Slaughter Cattle and Standards for Grades of Carcass Beef . Agricultural Marketing Services, USDA, Washington DC.

Ustuner, H., Yalcintan, H., Orman, A., Ardicli, S., Ekiz, B., Gencoglu, H. and Kandazoglu, O. (2017) Effects of Initial Fattening Age on Carcass Characteristics and Meat Quality in Simmental Bulls Imported from Austria to Turkey. South African Journal of Animal Science , 47, 194-201. https://doi.org/10.4314/sajas.v47i2.11

Warriss, P.D. (2000) Meat Science. CABI Publish, New York.

Wheeler, T.L., Candiff, L.V., Shackelford, S.D. and Koohmaraie, M. 2001. Characterization of biological types of cattle (cycle V): carcass and longissimus palatability. Journal of Animal Science. 79:1209-1222.

Workneh A, Ephrem G, Markos T, Yetnayet M, Rege JEO (2004). Farm Animal Biodiversity in Ethiopia: Status and Prospects, Current State of Knowledge on Characterization of Farm Animal Genetic Resources in Ethiopia. Proceedings of the 11th Annual conference of the Ethiopian Society of Animal Production (ESAP) held in Addis Ababa, Ethiopia, August 28-30, 2003. ESAP, Addis Ababa. 441pp.

Yesihak YM 2013 correlation between milk suckled and growth of calves of Ogaden cattle at one, three, and six months of age, east Ethiopia SpringerPlus 2013, 2:302 http://www.springerplus.com/content/2/1/302

Yesihak, M.Y. (2015) Beef Carcass Quality, Yield and Causes of Condemnation in Ethiopia. PhD Thesis, University of Pretoria, Pretoria.

Yesihak, M.Y. and Webb, E.C. (2014) Ethiopian Beef Carcass Characteristics. Afr ican Journal of Agricultural Research , 9, 3766-3775.

Yifat D, Bahilibi W, Desie S (2012). Reproductive Performance of Boran Cows at Tatesa Cattle Breeding Center. Adv. Biol. Res. 6(3):101-105.

Yifat D., Kelay B., Bekana M., Lobago F., Gustafsson H. and Kindahl H (2009). Study on reproductive performance of crossbred dairy cattle under smallholder conditions in and around Ziway, Ethiopia. Livestock Research for Rural Development 21 (6) 2009.

Yoseph M, Azage T, Alemu Y, Umunna N (2003). Evaluation of the General Farm Characteristics and Dairy Herd Structure in Urban and Peri-Urban Dairy Production System in the Addis Ababa Milk Shed. CGSpace A Repository of Agricultural Research Output.

Yoseph, M., Mengistu, U., Mohammed, Y.K. and Merga, B. (2011) Effect of Strategic Supplementation with Different Proportion of Agro-Industrial By-Products and Grass Hay on Body Weight Change and Carcass Characteristics of Tropical Ogaden Bulls (Bos indicus) Grazing Native Pasture. African Journal of Agricultural Research , 6, 825-833.

Zawadzki, F., Prado, I.N., Marques, J.A., Zeoula, L.M., Rotta, P.P., Sestari, B.B. and Rivaroli, D.C. (2011) Sodium Monensin or Propolis Extract in the Diets of Feedlot-Finished Bulls: Effects on Animal Performance and Carcass Characteristics. Journal of Animal and Feed Sciences, 20, 16-25. https://doi.org/10.22358/jafs/66153/2011

Zewdie w (2010). Livestock Production Systems in Relation with Feed Availability in the Highlands and Central Rift Valley, M.Sc. thesis submitted to the School of Animal and Range Sciences, School of Graduate Studies, Haramaya University, Ethiopia.